The Natural Hair Care Journey ... Top 5 Most-Asked Questions
By Laquita Thomas-Banks

Ordering information:
Discounts are available for quantity purchases. For details contact the author via BobeamNaturalProducts@gmail.com

Printed in the United States of America via CreateSpace.com
First Edition
Front/Back Cover Model: Laquita Thomas-Banks
ISBN 978-1507600610

Dedication

This book is dedicated to my mother and to the memory of my grandmother 'DeeDee' - my greatest cheerleaders.

Mom – my very first hair stylist. Her unique attention-grabbing weekend creations made me one of the popular girls in class on Monday mornings and she was the first person who bestowed on me the title of "Writer". Without your constant and persistent encouragement I would have never had the courage to live and follow my dreams.

My first outside-of-home "salon" experience was in DeeDee's kitchen. On special occasions she spent countless hours sweating, bent over my head pressing and curling my thick hair - I can still smell that hot comb, hear and feel the sizzling steam near my ears (and never once was burned) which resulted in bouncy curls and hair that stayed bone straight for weeks but always reverted right back – a true pioneer natural hair technician.

Table of Contents

Foreword

Let's face it. Historically, we've been taught that kinks, coils and nappy hair are unattractive, not sophisticated or appealing to the society at large or the opposite sex. Consequently, we've done everything under the sun to emulate the dominant culture's idea of what beautifully coiffed hair looks like.

Unfortunately, in this day of enlightenment, fake long hair, straight hair, bleached; light colored hair is still what some of us strive to have. It is difficult for some and impossible for others to embrace their God-given, naturally beautiful circles of tightly curled strands.

My father never allowed my mother to perm my sisters or my hair. She was not allowed to cut our hair either. My father forbade her to permanently alter what he called 'our crown and glory'.

Both my aunt and mother were hairstylists. Aunt Rose had salons in Philly and was licensed. Mother was a kitchen stylist who was self-taught. She used the straightening comb and hot curlers as her tools 'of torture' to tame her client's and her daughter's hair. Her routine hair dressing for the four of us sisters was....braids or ponytails unless there was a special occasion such as picture days at school, Easter, Christmas or Prom.

Having her business at home afforded her the 'luxury' of supplementing my father's income (as a truck driver) and be a stay at home mom. She was the perfect template for me to raise my family and stay in business. Learning that Madam C.J. Walker started her hair business from her home was confirmation for me as well.

While I hated to have my hair 'done' I somehow knew that straight was not for me. This book gives great dialog and example of 'this journey'. I tried to fit in because I didn't have any examples of anything else to do with my hair. Society, family and friends told me I would not be acceptable or taken seriously socially or in the business world if I did not conform to the status quo.

In 1965, I bucked and rebelled. I was one of the first teenagers in my neighborhood to sport an afro. Rebellious is what I was called. I accepted that title. Being a rebel has taken me to unimaginable heights and I am grateful and deeply humbled for this gift.

Rebelliousness gave me the courage to keep my salon open, in 1996, after the State Board of Cosmetology fined me and tried to shut me down. It pushed me to seek out other like-minded natural stylists (Cornrows & Co.) to wage and win the war against the ignorance that would keep me/and others from working and growing braid salons in Maryland.

My salon, Madam Walker's Braids received state exemption in 1997. I thank God that MWB has persevered and garnered much support. Along with my son, Shanti, we have maintained our natural hair salon, developed and taught the Art of Braiding for 12 years at Prince Georges Community College, and founded a non-profit foundation.

With the expert help and compassion of Laquita, who is a Board Chair of the foundation, we have awarded scholarships for women. Young people with passion, new ideas and new techniques for styling and caring for natural hair are a welcome addition to our roster of instructors at MWB Naturals.

Laquita is a graduate and certified natural hair stylist. She teaches a comprehensive course in product development at MWB Naturals. I can see why and how she should have written a book at this time. Her expertise and excellence in disciplines (hair, product development and journalism) make her a triple threat and a force to be reckoned with; hence, why this book is so important for not only clients but active, professional stylists as well.

Don't just peruse this book - jump in with both feet. Pay particular attention to Laquita's section on <u>10 Things Potential Natural Hair Wearers Should Know</u>. Her expert advice regarding her own hair journey is one that many of us can and do identify with - I know that I do. <u>How I Came to Embrace MY Hair Texture</u> is a chapter that we should share with our children. It's an interesting read and echoes all serious natural hair stylists.

Above all else, know the history of our craft. Pass along good lessons learned and proven by trial and error. Don't be a product junky. As Laquita says 'less is more' and water is your most valuable hair product.

Foreword *continued*

One of the most valuable things about this book is that it's more than a book; it's an experience in learning, sharing and communicating. As a practicing Natural Hair Care Stylist, certified in Maryland, Laquita has the experience and background to speak with authority on natural hair care and products. She has the educational know-how to do what this book is all about - knowing, loving and embracing your natural SELF inside and out.

Marci Walker-
Walker Enterprises... Madam Walker's Braids & Lockery – MWB Naturals – The S.E.L.F. Image Awards

Preface

I first decided to stop relaxing my hair over 20 years ago. I actually ventured on the natural hair journey twice before making the commitment to stay natural - as they say; the third time's the charm.

Throughout my natural hair journey, I have read several books, visited blogs, and natural hair online communities, watched hundreds of YouTube videos, and conducted tons of interviews, which have all provided me with valuable information on how to care for my hair and are all inspirations behind this book.

My favorite online community, Nappturality.com was the first online natural hair site that I discovered when I decided to wear my natural hair. I credit Nappturality.com and its creator, Patricia Gaines aka 'Dee', for not only keeping me on the path in my goal of maintaining healthy natural hair, but for also turning me into a self-proclaimed 'Natural Hair Ambassador'.

This book was also inspired by people that I have met riding on public transportation, standing in checkout lines in beauty supplies, grocery stores, etc. who either noticed my hair or I theirs and a conversation about natural hair was sparked. It is a condensed version of those conversations focusing on the most frequently asked questions and shared answers about hair care and the natural hair journey.

Ephesians 3:20, 21

The Transitioning Movement vs. The Black is Beautiful Movement

Over the past decade or more there has been a movement in the world of hair where women of all ages have decided to wear their hair natural. This 'transitioning movement' can be likened to a similar one that occurred over 40 years ago - the "Black is Beautiful" movement.

The "Black is Beautiful" movement, spiraling off of the Civil Rights Movement of the 1960s and early 70s, encouraged blacks to feel good about how they looked, and attempted to undue the notion that their natural traits were ugly. The movement is largely responsible for the popularity of the Afro. The movement asked that women and men stop straightening their hair and attempting to lighten or bleach their skin in attempt to reach the unattainable European-Americans' standard of beauty.

Now over 40 years later a "transitioning movement" is taking place. Similar to the ideals of "Black is Beautiful" movement, those who are transitioning from chemical straighteners to wearing their natural hair are undoing the notion that their natural traits (the hair growing from their head) is unattractive. And since this transitioning movement keeps growing stronger with more and more women everyday making the decision to stop using chemical straighteners, it does not seem to be a passing phase.

We all remember one of the most famous Afro wearing women of the "Black is Beautiful" era, Angela Davis. This former Black Panther gained nationwide notoriety when a weapon registered in her name was linked to the murder of Judge Harold Haley. Her arrest at the age of 26, and acquittal became one of the most famous trials in US History.

Well the "transitioning movement" may not have a famous historical trial as of yet, but not too long ago headlines detailed the stories of Laura Adiele, Timery Shante Nance and Isis Brantley's natural hair pat downs by the Transportation Security Administration, TSA, which caused quite a stir throughout the natural hair world and beyond.

The Transitioning Movement vs. The Black is Beautiful Movement
continued

Isis Brantley, a natural hair pioneer/activist was arrested in 1997 for braiding hair without a license in the state of Texas. At that time, there were no laws in the state that required braiders to be licensed, and many in the community saw the arrest as an attempt by the state to intimidate underground braiders and subject them to the same requirements as cosmetologists.

In 2004, Isis was able to get legislation to lower the cosmetology class hours from 1500 hours to 35 hours for those who want to solely practice natural hair care in the state of Texas. In 2007, she was grandfathered by the state of Texas as the first natural hair care expert and educator in the state. She also organized the 1st Natural Hair Parade & Festival - sponsored by Erykah Badu - held in Dallas, Texas.

Today transitioners and natural hair wearers, whether they be mothers, students, entertainers, activists, etc. are walking billboards shouting to the world and, most importantly, to the younger generation that natural hair is indeed beautiful. There are also several news shows as of late that have featured segments on transitioning and natural hair. MSNBC's Melissa Harris-Perry, who sports extension braids, had a panel of natural hair wearers on a show segment titled, "The Politics of Black Hair".

According to Black History.com the Black is Beautiful movement, "… gave a generation of Blacks the courage to feel good about who they were and how they looked. This reaffirmation carried over into today's society, where many Black people, particularly Black women, are more proud of their hair, faces, and bodies than other races in terms of self-esteem."

Therefore, the "transitioning movement" can be viewed as one that was birthed from the "Black is Beautiful" movement. It is something that I believe will continue on from our generation well into the future. I can even imagine one day " transitioning " being a term of the past or rarely used. Young girls growing up will have so many beautiful images of natural hair around them that they wouldn't ever dream of changing the hair texture they were born with.

Characteristics of the Natural Hair Wearer

There have been many stereotypical definitions of the "Natural Hair Wearer" - militant, Afro-wearing, 100% natural, no weaves or extensions, no chemicals whatsoever inside or out, vegan, and the list goes on and on. But in reality the description is just like all stereotypes - a conventional, formulaic, and oversimplified conception (definition a la Webster).

Within the past decade, there has been a resurgence of natural hair wearers. This resurgence is similar to the rise of natural hair wearers in the 60s during the Black Power and Black is Beautiful Movement, where both men and women embraced their natural hair making the Afro iconic.

Not only are natural hair wearers sporting Afros, but both men and women are donning everything from artistic braid, twist and loc styles, to textured curly and free form kinky styles as well as precision designed barber cuts, showcasing their chemical straightener -free natural hair.

To state the obvious, no, not all naturals are vegan or vegetarians, and many could care less whether the person standing in line in front of them at the check out counter, next to them on the bus or a coworker has a perm or relaxer or sports a bone straight weave or wig, and most times will even compliment a straight style on the color or cut.

Many natural hair wearers have added color to their hair and thus are not 100% free of chemicals, but feel that as long as the added color does not alter the curl pattern of their hair, it is still to be considered as natural. Now there are some 100% free natural hair wearers, but likewise most embrace their color-treated natural brothers and sisters just the same.

Who are these natural hair wearers? Again, although natural hair wearers are often generalized as one group each one of these women and men are unique. They are your next door neighbors, athletes, they head and own businesses, are parents, students, mothers, politicians, actresses, musicians and artists from all walks of life.

Therefore, natural hair styles can be spotted not only on city or suburban streets, but everywhere from school campuses, board rooms, on the big screen at movie theaters, sports arenas, fashion runways to concert halls. Likewise, more than one style or technique can be spotted on a single head i.e. cornrows with frohawks, flat-twists with curly ends, or fros and locs with shaved designs.

Characteristics of the Natural Hair Wearer *continued*

Just as the definition of a natural hair wearer is broad, natural hair wearers have their own definitions of what "natural" means to them. Many compare it to how some define Hip-Hop - a culture, a movement associated with style/fashion, a state of mind.

Ayo Fashola, Authentic Style Coach™ sums it up well. "Until you can deal with being authentic within, how you wear your hair or the term you call it is irrelevant. I consider myself natural because I have total clarity on who I am and my identity, which I call sensuous cultivated.

The sensuous part of me represents anything lush, sexy and that stimulates the senses, highly feminine and vibrant. My own natural hair allows me to express this specific part of me, anything else and I'll be contradicting my genuine identity.

The cultivated part of my style statement allows me to always maintain a level of grace and refinement, so my hair will always be done, well conditioned and treated with the utmost love and care so that my hair can cultivate (grow). I'm in sync and in tune with who I am, so I'm ready to call myself...natural."

10 Things Potential Natural Hair Wearers Should Know

When you embark on the natural hair journey, you will come across lots of information to guide you along the way. For those who are contemplating wearing their hair natural or for those who are in the process of transitioning, here are ten potential things you should know.

1. Your hands are the best styling tools.

2. Natural hair thrives when well moisturized and conditioned.

3. Water is a great detangler and moisturizer.

4. Using an oil or pomade on wet hair seals in moisture.

5. Less is better when it comes to applying products.

6. You'll have to experiment with products, even if they are natural, because what works for someone else may not work for you.

7. Braiding or banding both help to stretch natural hair, therefore no heat is required.

8. Lemon juice, apple cider vinegar, baking soda and brown sugar can be used as scalp cleansers.

9. Protective styles – those that require less everyday manipulation, aid in overall hair health.

10. Straw-sets, updos, chignons, pin curls and spiral curls can all be achieved with natural hair, so the styles are limitless.

II

Some of the Most Asked Hair Questions Answered...

A. How Did I Get My Hair Like That?

This is definitely one of the most asked questions about my hair, and oddly enough I feel people ask me this question when my hair is not looking its best.

A freshly untwisted twist-out with a ton of my scalp showing because I didn't want to separate the twists fully to avoid frizz, an old bun that I have meticulously smoothed back into place with Shea butter, or a still fresh (wet) wash and go – are the styles that get the most attention.

The styles that I spend hours at a time on – intricately parted flat twists or cornrowed styles - barely get a quick glance. Oceans of slick backed waves, elongated bouncy spirals and curly-q curls are definitely eye-catching but don't come easy for all hair types. And although most of us know this, we still ask the question, "How do I get MY hair to do that?"

And in all honesty, in the beginning of my hair journey I asked the same question.

Chasing the Curly Look

In the beginning of my natural hair journey, I found myself gravitating toward products promising touchable, elongated, bouncy, curly ringlets - especially those claiming to work on '4-type' kinkier hair texture. Although I knew for a fact that some hair textures just don't form the perfect curly Q elongated curls, and that not everything worked for everybody, I just couldn't stop myself from trying those products.

When I came across such products and their before and after pictures along with accompanying testimonies, I would browse through the before and after pictures over and over, focusing on the 'before' shots that depicted models with hair texture closest to mine.

After examining each and every curl in the 'after' shots and deciding that the curls actually 'do' look touchable, elongated and bouncy, I would make my move. I'd click on the 'add to shopping cart' link and anxiously await the arrival of my product. "Oooo wait until product 'ABC' arrives, I am going to post pictures and everyone will wonder what I used," I would think to myself.

When the fateful day - which always seemed like it took forever - arrived and I would see my package sitting outside of my front door, I didn't hesitate to dive right in. And almost every time, as I was applying product 'ABC' I could immediately see results. My kinks were stretching, curls were forming and there was shine for days!

And likewise, almost every time as product 'ABC' started to dry the elongated curls either; A) slowly began to shrink, matt together and no longer looked defined, B) the shine began to fade leaving behind a cloudy film, C) Shrunken curls remained, but my hair felt like old leaves - dry and crunchy, or D) the curls remained elongated, but were hard and 'frozen' in place - nowhere near touchable or bouncy.

For some reason, no matter how many times I experienced one, or all of the above after using curling products I still chased after them. I didn't even care about the length - I longed for what appeared to be 'wake-up-n-go' curls - sans re-wetting, or by way of twist-outs/braid-outs or straw sets, etc. - that Sydney T. Poitier circa Grindhouse hair!

Chasing the Curly Look *continued*

Now, I'm not saying I didn't like my hair texture - I loved that I could wear a big afro puff one day and bouncy full braid-out the next, with only the use of water and a moisturizer, and had onlookers wondering if I wore hairpieces, but I also wanted those curls. In essence, I wanted it all - the curls, the kinks, everything! I felt I was the only one with this impossible dream, and often thought is, "it 'really' impossible?"

Back in those days, I could've just sat idle and been satisfied with the versatility of my texture, but I always thought what if by chance I stumble upon product 'ABC2.0' that actually did what it says it will do? I will touch and swing my curls, while posting my pics, spread the word and be celebrated by fellow '4-type' hair textures everywhere! I would think, "Ah - that will be the good life".

How I Came to Embrace MY Hair Texture

During my transitioning journey, I also remember watching videos and visiting hair journey blogs and Ooing and Aahing over silky smooth curl patterns. I couldn't wait until my transition was over so my very own silky smooth curls could be unleashed. Like so many other natural hair enthusiasts I think I had the mindset of going natural to go curly.

Throughout my transition, I slowly began to notice that the texture of my hair didn't appear to be the same as those I had been drooling over on the blogs and videos. But I kept my eyes on the prize and just figured with a little "training" my texture could be whipped into shape.

I figured it was the products that these ladies were using that produced these silky smooth curls. So, as stated previously, I began my product scavenger hunt. After piling on tons of products - and unbeknownst to me at the time actually weighing down my curls – I realized that the products weren't helping me achieve my goal of silky smooth curls.

Even though I stood in the bathroom mirror disappointed, broke, and white-headed with product running down my face I still didn't put two and two together. I reasoned, "It's not the products that will unleash my curls; I must find the perfect techniques or routine."

So after studying routines and techniques which included co-washes, CWC – condition, wash, condition, L.O.C. methods – liquid, oil, cream, sleeping with shower caps on – baggie method, etc. – you know all of the cool natural hair terms and acronyms - I was confident my goal of silky smooth curls would be met.

Well I must admit that after following these routines my hair was softer and super moisturized and I even spotted a few more defined coils here and there. Nonetheless, I still didn't achieve my silky smooth curls. And even then I decided to experiment a bit more switching up different products along with these techniques, but again to no avail.

I had to finally face the music; piling on products and strictly following other people's routines did not yield the silky smooth curls I had envisioned. What was I to do? Well, first off, I decided to give my hair and myself a much needed break. Chasing after a particular curl pattern was not only exhausting but stressful.

How I Came to Embrace MY Hair Texture *continued*

Out of money, stressed and exhausted, I decided to simply wash, condition and add a little oil or pomade to my hair and just let it be. On occasion, I added a few flat twists in the front, put on a headband or hair clips, but that was the extent of my routine. It was short, sweet and simple. I actually began to love my not-so-smooth kinky coils and to my surprise other people liked them as well.

I began to get compliments from friends, family members and strangers on how nice my hair looked and inquiries on what I did to keep it looking so healthy and shiny.

I was actually thrilled when a few people even asked if I had put a texturizer in my hair. These compliments came after only a few weeks of my low product and simple routine.

I realized I had spent months buying tons of products and following other people's routines with the unattainable goal of achieving THEIR curl pattern. Even though my kinky coils were not the "smooth and silky" ones I coveted, they were and are still beautiful as well.

So for all those who are transitioning and/or newly natural learn from my experience. Become familiar with your own curl pattern/hair texture. Learn what your hair likes/dislikes and develop a routine that will help your hair grow healthy and strong.

Through months of stressful trial and error, I learned that growing a head full of healthy hair should be the primary goal versus the unrealistic one of attaining someone else's curl pattern. It was not only a valuable lesson, but one in which I learned to embrace my hair texture.

B. How Do I Keep My Hair Moisturized?

Moisturizing 101 (Summer/Winter Months)

Keeping your hair moisturized in the summer may seem like a hard task, but it's actually pretty simple. The best moisturizer for natural hair is WATER. I've found that natural hair loves water.

Of course, if you spend time outside in the summer heat your hair will become dry. The best way to combat this dryness is with a refreshing spritz of water.

Water mixed with a little soluble essential oil, like lavender oil and a water based conditioner will keep your hair from feeling dry and brittle, and your scalp moisturized. Adding the lavender oil or a little of your favorite scent will also keep your hair smelling great.

If you are wearing braided or twist styles you will be able to spritz directly onto your scalp - in-between the parts, and will be able to spritz at least twice daily without affecting your hairstyle.

If you are wearing a 'loose' style, like a twist out or afro, and do not necessarily want to wet your hair, use an applicator bottle to moisten your scalp daily, or if you braid your loose style at night spritz after braiding. Be sure to follow with a light oil or pomade to seal in the moisture after you spritz.

You can find a variety of purse-sized and bigger spray bottles in your local drug or grocery store, usually no more than $0.99. For extra pampering you can fill your bottle with spring or filtered water, with your added e/o and/or favorite scent, and conditioner, and keep it stored in your fridge for a cool, refreshing mist right after you come in from a long day of being out in the summer heat. This bottle can also be used to refill your purse-sized bottle.

Be sure to refresh your purse-sized bottle each morning with a fresh batch. You can also add a little sage oil to preserve your spritz if you are going to keep it longer than five days; lemon juice and/or a drop of honey will also do the trick.

Moisturizing 101 *continued*

If you use honey, be sure to let the mixture sit for a few days - so the honey can fully dissolve in the water to prevent stickiness (and with all mixes, shake well before using). Even if you use a preservative, I suggest that you refresh your spritz every two weeks.

Winter Months

Likewise keeping your hair moisturized during the winter months is not as hard as it may seem.

Some may shy away from moisturizing their hair in the winter because of the obvious reason - it's cold. But, keeping your hair moisturized in the colder months is just as important as keeping it moisturized in the warmer ones.

Dry scalp is common in the cold weather or if you have high central heating because both can affect the amount of moisture in the scalp, therefore you must keep your hair and scalp moisturized.

The most effective way to moisturize your hair and scalp is with water. The simplest way to moisturize your hair and scalp is by either running your hands under the faucet for a few seconds then running them through your hair, or again using a spritz bottle to lightly dampen your hair.

And remember, right after doing either of those methods; apply a little oil or pomade to seal in the moisture.

Of course, in the colder months you may not want to spritz or dampen your hair right before heading outside. To avoid having to go outside with damp hair moisturize and seal your hair at night.

Your hair doesn't have to be soaking wet to be moisturized, lightly dampened or spritzed is more than enough. Doing this three or four times a week will ensure that your hair stays moisturized.

This routine also helps to smooth frizzy hair and fly-aways and give older protective styles such as braided updos, cornrows, or twists a fresh look.

After your moisture and seal routine, simply tie on a satin or silk scarf (not too tight) and in the morning your style will look refreshed.

Moisturizing 101 *continued*

Another thing you can do to keep your hair moisturized in the winter months is pre-shampoo - aka- pre-poo. Do a pre-poo with oil before washing to provide added moisture. After taking down a style in preparation to wash or 20 minutes before washing, just rub some oil through your hair from roots to ends.

You can then cover your hair with a plastic cap and wash in the morning, or hop in the shower letting the steam work with the oil like a hot oil treatment then wash.

In the winter months also make sure you use moisturizing shampoos and conditioners. You may also want to deep condition more often during the colder months as well. You can add more moisture to your conditioners by mixing in a little oil.

As you are about to apply your conditioner pour a quarter sized amount of oil such as olive oil in your hands along with the conditioner and apply the mixture from roots to tips. If you do this on soaking wet hair, you can even use a regular conditioner and leave this mixture in since the conditioner will be diluted.

Be sure to pay extra care to the ends of your hair in the winter months. Dry, split ends cause breakage while moisturized ends are more pliable and retain length.

Protect your ends by wearing silk or satin scarves around your shoulders to keep your ends from rubbing against wool coats and cotton sweaters.

Make sure that the hats you wear have a silk or satin lining or wear a silk/satin scarf underneath. Cotton absorbs moisture and also snags your hair, therefore at night use a silk/satin scarf, bonnet or pillow case.

One final tip when it comes to helping your hair retain moisture is to whenever possible stay away from high heat, styling tools i.e. hand-held dryers, flat irons and curling irons.

Challenge yourself to avoid these things altogether in the winter season. Preferably, air dry your hair, and blot with a towel. But if you must use heat to dry, use a bonnet-dryer on low heat.

Following one or more of these steps will ensure that your hair will be moisturized throughout the summer and winter season and all year round.

L.O.C./L.C.O. Moisturizing Methods for Dry Hair

During your natural hair journey if you find that no matter what you do to your hair it seems to always feel dry you should try the L.O.C. or L.C.O. method to keep your hair moisturized.

L.O.C. is an acronym for Liquid, Oil, Cream and L.C.O. is an acronym for Liquid, Cream, Oil. Both of these methods are good to try if you are experiencing dry hair. They both require layering on products to keep your hair well moisturized.

The first step in both methods "L" is applying liquid to your hair. I find that the best liquid for my hair is water. Some apply a liquid-based moisturizing leave-in conditioner. So for those, the "L" in both methods stands for leave-in.

But either way, the first step is to wet your hair with a liquid-based product. You can either wash your hair or use a spray bottle to spritz your hair with water, leave-in conditioner or a mixture of both.

The second step in the L.O.C. method is an oil - the "O". With this method, after you apply your liquid, you apply a light layer of oil to seal in the moisture. The last step in the L.O.C. method is the "C" - cream.

After applying oil, you apply a light layer of a creamy product to seal in moisture. The creamy product can be a butter-based cream like a curling pudding or even hair milk type product. If you used just water as your liquid, your "C" in this step can even be a leave-in conditioner.

Now the second and third steps in the L.C.O. method are reversed. The second step is "C" – the cream, and the third step "O" is oil. Some people find that applying the oil last acts as a sealant for both the liquid and cream, and that it keeps their hair moisturized longer. It's best to try both methods to see which one works best for your hair.

You can experiment with products within the methods as well. For example, a styling product with a little hold like an alcohol-free gel can be used in place of the creamy product "C" in both methods depending on the type of hairstyle you are wearing.

L.O.C./L.C.O. Moisturizing Methods for Dry Hair *continued*

Both methods are ideal for wash-and-go styles. They both can be done at night as overnight moisturizing treatment methods as well. After following the steps in either method, simply cover your hair with a plastic shower cap before going to bed and in the morning just rinse your hair and style.

Likewise, both methods can both be done as monthly deep conditioning methods with braided, straight and loose styles as well. Again, simply follow the steps in either method, and then cover your hair with a plastic shower cap either overnight or for 30 minutes, rinse and style.

No matter which method you decide to use you will notice an immediate difference in your hair. Keeping your hair well moisturized will help lessen breakage and split ends and result in length retention.

Bedtime Moisturizing Hair Care Routines

We all know that covering our hair at night keeps styles from looking crazy in the morning. Using a silk/satin scarf or bonnet or sleeping on a silk/satin pillowcase also protects the ends of your hair, as well as keeps it from being snagged and pulled out by cotton pillowcases or scarves.

I love doing overnight pre-shampoo treatments, aka pre-poos, or conditioning and moisturizing treatments (like the L.O.C./L.C.O. methods mentioned earlier) and the baggy method. I use oil for pre-poos.

The main purpose of pre-shampoo treatments is to get rid of build-up, especially if you are heavy-handed with products at times like I am. Doing pre-poos also help wash days go faster because you will not have to lather over and over again when you wash your hair.

Although some pre-poo with conditioner, I like to use oil. I like using oil on water-spritzed hair as I take down my old style and detangle. As I detangle, I put my hair in loose braids and massage the oil in my scalp and down the length of each braid.

Massaging the oil in my scalp and down each braid helps to loosen up build-up and also seal in moisture from the spritzing. After I complete my entire head, I cover my head with a plastic shower cap for the night then wash in the morning.

Again, this cuts down my wash time because I don't need tons of lather. Washing my hair with the braids in makes detangling easier as well and results in less breakage.

Now for those who like a more scientific explanation of how pre-poos are beneficial, in an Q&A article written by CurlyNikki (of CurlyNikki.com) for Essence.com she stated, "Pre-poo treatments greatly reduce hygral fatigue -the expanding and contracting of hair as water enters and exits - and help maintain the structural integrity of the cuticle and cortex."

Bedtime Moisturizing Hair Care Routines *continued*

For more scientific information on hygral fatigue, visit TheNaturalHairHavenBloom.com and check out her post –"Does your hair have hygral fatigue?"

Also, oil dissolves oil. Again in scientific lingo: Oil is made up of carbon atoms bonded to hydrogen atoms forming hydrocarbon chains, which makes them non-polar. Polar substances will only dissolve polar substances, i.e., like dissolves like.

Another way to treat your hair at night is the baggy method. The baggy method can be done on wet or dry hair. The process involves using a mix of oil and conditioner to keep your ends moisturized in between washes.

Covering either your entire head or just your bun, puff or ponytail with a plastic shower cap, plastic wrap or small plastic bag after moisturizing seals in moisture, which results in length retention because your ends will not break due to dryness.

Unlike the pre-poo, after doing the baggy method you do not wash your hair. On dry hair, apply a water-based leave-in conditioner or cream mixed with a little oil to your ends then cover with your cap, Saran Wrap or bag.

For those with longer hair, you can either put your hair in one puff, bun or ponytails -plaited or twisted and rolled into a bun - then apply your mix and cover (you can use elastic metal-free bands to secure plastic bags to your bun).

On wet hair you can apply an oil or butter-based conditioning product. Again, the purpose of the baggy method is to seal in moisture in-between washes, which will result in less breakage, due to dry and brittle ends, and length retention.

C. How Do I Get My Hair To Grow?

Resisting Hair Growth Remedies

As our hair grows on average a half an inch a month, or six inches a year, barring any health disparities, to say that transitioners must have patience is an understatement.

I know for me, when I was on the transitioning journey – for the third time mind you – I would just drool (I sure did a lot of drooling) over photos of women sporting their natural hair and couldn't bare the wait until my hair was chemical free. I remember taking down my transition styles each month with anticipation, excited to see if by some miracle my new growth had grown over its usual 1/2 inch.

I was super excited when I came across Mane 'n Tail – now this wasn't the Mane 'n Tail they have on the store shelves today made for humans – this was the original straight from the farm bottle with directions telling me I could use it to condition and clean my hooves as well. I'll tell you I went through who knows how many bottles of that shampoo. But in the end I had the same results 1/2 inch of growth a month.

Nowadays, Mane 'n Tail has an entire line of products made for human hair and I have come across many testimonies stating how it actually helps people's hair to grow. Over the years of my natural hair journey I have also stumbled upon other types of hair growth remedies or treatments.

With one quick search on the internet, you will come across various posts from at home growth remedies such as using garlic and onion juice on your scalp which are purported to work due to their high sulfur levels, to using a mixture of Cayenne pepper and castor oil or even vodka to grow your tresses.

Cayenne pepper has actually been used as a home remedy to grow hair for centuries. It is said to help improve blood circulation. The most bizarre remedy I have come across is the use of a bull semen conditioning treatment to grow hair, which to me sounds like an extreme act of desperation!

Resisting Hair Growth Remedies *continued*

Now, while the at home remedies such as onions, garlic and cayenne pepper may not have any foreseen side effects, I would like to alert those seeking growth remedies to be cautious about using topical ointments such as Monistat 7 – yes the vaginal cream – and supplements. Be sure to consult a doctor before taking prenatal pills and/or biotin.

Also be cautions about using Monistat 7 or Minoxidil aka Rogaine. Although there are several YouTube videos that show great results with Monistat 7. There are also possible side effects such as Migraine headaches, tenderness/burning and extreme shedding once you stop using it.

There are also a great deal of testimonies of how the use of Minoxidil results in hair growth, but just as many more that state once people stop using it, just as with Monistat 7, they experience hair loss. Side effects also include dizziness, irregular heart beat and chest pain.

Now as a side note those of us who have sought out and maybe even tried hair growth remedies are not alone, and actually hair growth remedies are nothing new. In fact, Egyptians, Greeks and Romans used hair growth remedies, with ingredients ranging from pigeon droppings to animal fat. But all in all, to be on the safe side a healthy diet, exercise and patience are the best remedies for side effect-free healthy hair growth.

Clean Scalp Equals Healthy Hair

There are many people who believe that a dirty scalp is the key to hair growth, but in fact the opposite is true. Washing your hair actually prevents scalp disorders and diseases. Our scalp attracts and retains dirt when it is not routinely washed. This can result in clogged hair follicles and thinning and dry hair.

Keeping your scalp clean keeps it free from oil, dirt, dead skin cell and product build-up which can clog hair follicles and prevent hair growth, even causing hair loss. Keeping your scalp clean and moisturized will stop itching, prevent scalp damage and hair loss. Therefore, a clean scalp equals healthy hair.

Washing your hair also prevents sebum (scalp's natural oils) from collecting in the scalp's pores and hair follicles which can lead to scalp problems such as overactive sebaceous glands. When sebaceous glands are out of balance, this can result in either an overproduction or underproduction of sebum.

When there is too much sebum, it will eventually harden and hinder hair growth, resulting in thinning hair and eventual hair loss. When there is too little sebum, hair becomes dry and brittle which also results in hair loss.

Washing your hair/scalp with chemical-free products and with those that contain essential oils also helps to balance your scalp's natural oils.

For those with longer hair (past ear length) a great way to wash your hair is in sections. Washing and conditioning your hair in sections versus piling it up on top of your head will prevent it from tangling and matting. This really helps when transitioning and having to deal with two different textures of hair – new growth and straight ends.

I personally do not like wash days, but washing my hair in sections helps the process go smoothly.

Retaining Length – Detangling/Washing

First of all, to minimize breakage when washing and detangling make sure you designate time to wash and detangle your hair. Set aside a specific day to wash your hair. By doing this, you will be able to take your time and will not feel rushed. This will result in less pulling and breaking.

I found one of the best ways to wash natural hair is to separate it into sections, depending on how long your hair is, you may be able to loosely braid each section before washing.

Preparation – As stated earlier before washing I detangle and 'pre-poo' with natural oils such as olive oil, rice bran oil, grapeseed oil, etc. After taking down my previous style, I detangle using my hands first, and then use a wide tooth comb.

As a pre-poo I massage my scalp with oil, sort of like a hot-oil treatment without the heat. This can also be done with heated oil for an actual hot-oil treatment, but to ensure you don't burn your scalp sit your oil in a bowl of boiling water for a few minutes to warm the oil or put on a shower cap and/or shower to let the steam from the shower do the heating.

After massaging my scalp with the oil, I braid my hair into six to eight loose braids, being careful not to braid too tight or close to the roots so I am able to wash my scalp. And again, to cut down on time spent during this routine I do my pre-poo and braiding at night.

Routine...

As you braid or section your hair, use a spray bottle filled with water and/or essential oil and lightly spray and gently detangle each section with your hands or a wide tooth comb if necessary.

During this step, you can pre-poo as well by massaging your scalp with an oil, or spray in a conditioner rinse which can be a conditioner diluted with water and your favorite oil.

Next, while your hair is sectioned or braided, wet your hair. Add a small amount of cleanser to each section and massage your scalp with the pads of you fingers and work/squeeze the suds through to the ends. Continue this until each section has been washed, then rinse your entire head with cool water.

Retaining Length – Detangling/Washing *continued*

After rinsing you can now add your conditioner. Work the conditioner into each section gently massaging from ends to roots. For deep conditioning, put on a plastic shower cap/bag or heating cap for 10 to 30 mins.

With the conditioner still in your hair, gently detangle each section (if braided, unbraid and detangle) using your fingers first then, if necessary, a wide tooth comb starting from the ends moving up to the roots. Once all sections have been detangled, gently rinse your hair with cool water. After your initial rinse, you can follow with a clarifying rinse such as an ACV or tea rinse as your final rinse.

Do not ring out your hair nor squeeze dry with a towel. Gently pat dry so your hair is not dripping wet, being careful not to roughly rub the towel against your hair. While your hair is damp you can also apply a leave-in conditioner and moisturizer.

Let your hair air dry or style while still damp. If you are planning on wearing a wash-n-go, after moisturizing while your hair is still wet add your alcohol-free styling aid or curl product being careful not to disturb the pattern of your curls, so they will keep their form as your hair dries.

This method may seem long and tedious, but the results are wonderful – less breakage and length retention :o)

Preventing Split Ends

Split ends, scientifically known as Trichoptilosis, happens when the hair's protective cuticle has been stripped away from the ends, causing a splitting of the hair shaft giving it a feathery appearance.

Avoiding trims, excessive brushing, heat, elastic bands, hair extensions, towel drying and even dry scalp are all causes of split ends. There is no 'cure' for split ends, the only way to get rid of them is to cut them off.

The ends of your hair are very important. Dry, split ends cause breakage while moisturized ends are more pliable and retain length. Some people shy away from trimming their ends because they do not want to lose length.

But keep in mind that split ends cause the hair to split all the way up to the scalp, which will result in you having to get a major cut. Split ends should be cut at least 1 inch above the split.

Another good way to prevent split ends, along with moisturizing, is adding 'dusting' of your ends to your hair routine. I would describe dusting as cutting off less than an inch of your ends.

When your ends start to feel crunchy, or you hear popping when you detangle, or start to see tiny hairs in the sink that are not old shed hairs (with white bulbs at the tips) these are signs that you may need to 'dust' your ends.

The easiest way to trim/dust your own ends is when your hair is in box braids or twists. Simply cut a little (about a half inch or less) off the ends of each twist or braid.

To protect your ends, get in the routine of moisturizing them during the week. Use oils such as Shea butter, castor oil, olive oil or almond oil to protect your ends.

Conditioning after shampooing (rinse with cool water to close your hair cuticle), detangling with conditioner, and adding a monthly deep conditioner to your hair care routine also help prevent split ends, as well as avoiding heat, air drying whenever possible, and keeping your hair moisturized.

Preventing Split Ends *continued*

Wearing 'protective' styles, such as braids, cornrows or twists are also helpful in protecting your ends. Cotton absorbs moisture and also snags your hair, therefore at night use a silk/satin scarf, bonnet or pillow case.

Consider Ayurvedic Natural Hair Care

Ayurveda is a holistic approach to health that is designed to help people live long, healthy, and well-balanced lives. The term Ayurveda is taken from the Sanskrit words ayus, meaning life or lifespan, and veda, meaning knowledge. It has been practiced in India for at least 5,000 years. The basic principle of Ayurveda is to prevent and treat illness with natural herbal remedies and first and foremost by maintaining balance in the body, mind, and consciousness through proper diet, and lifestyle.

We all know that poor diet, illness, lack of proper hygiene, and nutritional deficiencies can all affect the hair and cause various problems. Many are taking an Ayurvedic approach to maintaining healthy hair.

A Quick lesson in Ayurveda

In Ayurveda, doshas are the functional intelligences within the body mind complex; they are the energies that make things happen within an organism. There are three dosha predominant constitutions; **Vata**, **Pitta**, and **Kapha**, where two doshas are equally or nearly equally predominant (Vata-Pitta, Pitta-Kapha and Vata-Kapha; and one tridoshic Prakruti with all three doshas equally prominent Vata-Pitta-Kapha)

Everyone has Vata, Pitta, and Kapha, but usually one or two are dominant in a particular person. Stress and an unhealthy diet are among the things that can disturb the doshas balance.

Vata is the energy of movement. It is the energy that controls bodily functions associated with motion including blood circulation, breathing, blinking and heartbeat. When it is balanced creativity and vitality are present. When Vata is not balanced, this produces fear and anxiety.

Pitta is the energy of digestion and metabolism. It is the energy that controls the body's metabolic systems, including digestion, absorption, nutrition, and temperature. When Pitta is balanced contentment and intelligence are present. When it is not balanced anger and even ulcers arise.

Kapha is the energy of lubrication and structure. It is the energy that controls growth in the body. This energy supplies water to all body parts moisturizes the skin and maintains the immune system. When Kapha is balanced, love and forgiveness are present. When it is not balanced, it results in insecurity and envy.

Consider Ayurvedic Natural Hair Care *continued*

Ayurveda Holistic Hair Care

Ayurvedic Herbs

Shikakai
A natural astringent and gentle cleanser, shikakai is referred to as "fruit for the hair". It helps to clear dandruff, is a natural hair conditioner and has a mild pH.

Aritha
Known as soapnut, it is a natural shampoo for oily hair.

Tulsa
Known as the Holy Basil and regarded as a kind of "elixir of life". It is a natural cleanser and good for oily hair. It protects from hair loss and premature graying.

Neem
Good for dry itchy sensitive skin and dandruff. It prevents hair loss, dryness and nourishes the scalp.

Brahmi
Helps with hair thinning and relieves itchy scalp. It is an excellent product in clearing dandruff.

Amla
Known as the Indian Gooseberry, it is a natural source of vitamin C. It is a natural astringent which works on both hair and skin. It is a great conditioning herb. It helps to prevent scalp infection while controlling premature graying of the hair and promoting hair growth.

Lemon Peel
Cleanser and astringent, helps to balance the skin's natural oil.

Sandalwood
Most sacred herbs of Ayurveda. It is antimicrobial (capable of destroying or inhibiting the growth of disease-causing microorganisms), antiseptic, astringent.
It has hydrating properties, making it an ideal cleanser for gentle, sensitive skin. Good for dry hair and scalp.

Consider Ayurvedic Natural Hair Care *continued*

When it comes to hair care, the Ayurvedic practice of keeping the doshas balanced play a key role in maintaining healthy hair. Along with the obvious things, like moisturizing, conditioning, protecting your ends, minimizing the use of heat, etc, incorporate the following Ayurvedic steps to ensure healthy hair.

1. Start with a nutritious diet. Eat lots of leafy green vegetables, fresh fruits and nuts - avoid caffeinated drinks, spicy, fried and greasy food. Foods such as white sesame seeds, whole grains, dates and raisins, fresh yogurt, bean sprouts, and healthy fats such as olive oil, are great for overall hair health.

Cook with spices that enhance digestion and purify body tissues: turmeric, black pepper, fenugreek, coriander and cumin which is digestion-enhancing (balancing **Pitta**). Also, add vitamins and supplements to your diet.

2. Make weekly hair and scalp massages part of your hair care routine which nourish your hair and scalp and enhance circulation (balancing **Vata**) - olive oil will do the trick. You can also infuse your oil with herbs by steeping a tea bag filled with chamomile, hibiscus etc, in hot oil for a few hours then using the cooled mixture to massage your scalp and/or use it as a hot-oil treatment.

3. Follow a regular cleansing routine (balancing **Kapha**). Whether you do this daily, weekly or bi-weekly, a clean, build-up free scalp is one of the major keys to healthy hair. Remember, wash your scalp with the pads of your fingers not your nails and do a final rinse with cool water. Also, remember to clean your hair tools as well, soaking brushes and combs in boiled water and/or shampoo regularly helps to get rid of dead skin cells, oils and dirt.

4. Balance all three doshas, **Pitta**, **Vata**, and **Kapha** by managing stress, and getting plenty of sleep. Stress can lead to hair loss and sleep deprivation is a form of stress. Emotional or physical stress related to a death in the family, pregnancy, severe weight loss or surgery pushes large numbers of growing hairs into a resting phase resulting in hair loss called telogen effluvium. Although it can take months, this type of hair loss grows back when the emotional or physical stress is resolved.

Consider Ayurvedic Natural Hair Care *continued*

For some, intense stress may trigger a type of hair loss called alopecia areata. With this type of hair loss, white blood cells attack the hair follicle which stops hair growth and within weeks, the affected hair falls out. This type of hair loss usually starts as a small round patch, but may eventually spread to the whole scalp, and sometimes to body hair as well. The hair generally grows back, but the cycle may repeat itself.

Keeping a journal, making time for hobbies, going for walks and taking long baths, are just a few of the ways to manage and/or reduce stress. Try practicing Yoga and meditation, which are the primary Ayurvedic treatments for stress. By making these things a part of your lifestyle, you will see a great improvement in the health of your hair and overall health.

Wearing Protective Styles for Growth Retention

Protective 'low manipulation' hairstyles reduce the amount of hair breakage, aid in length retention and protect against split ends. Braids, cornrows, twists, buns, updos, wigs and even headwraps can be worn to protect your hair and can be worn for long periods of time with little to no manipulation.

I embarked on a journey of wearing my hair in protective styles for an entire year. From August of '08 to August of '09 I solely wore protective styles which helped me achieve much healthier hair and I retained about five inches of growth.

The use of silk/satin scarves or bonnets is great for preserving styles, but for some reason they manage to jump off the moment we lay our heads on the pillow. The next best thing is satin pillow cases.

Satin pillow cases help preserve hairstyles and are a great backup plan for runaway scarves and bonnets. Also make sure you take out all bows and barrettes before bedtime, and if your hair is long enough for a ponytail, put the braids and/or twists in a loose ponytail with metal free elastics.

In-between styling to combat some of the frizziness and/or for moisturizing during the week, lightly spray your hair with a leave-in conditioning spray, then add a little pomade or oil to seal in the moisture then tie hair down with a silk/satin scarf. (This can be done two to three times a week for moisturizing).

With cornrows or flat twists, you can also use a soft bristled brush or a baby brush, to brush flat loose hair coming from the cornrows/flat twists in the direction the hair is braided or twisted, before tying on the scarf.

This can be done before bedtime or 30 minutes to an hour before you leave the house and really refreshes flat styles. If you find it necessary to wash braided or twisted styles before the second week, just use your designated styling day for a quick wash.

When washing loose/hanging braids or twists you can braid sections together or band them before washing. This will help with frizz and unraveling. Braided twists or single braids can also be unraveled after they dry to give the style a new crinkled/wavy look.

Wearing Protective Styles for Growth Retention *continued*

To preserve cornrows or flat twists while washing, you can put a stocking cap over the style and wash – being careful not to disturb the cornrows or twists, concentrating on your scalp. Leave-in conditioners can also be added after washing and remember to add your pomade or oil to seal in moisture.

D. How Do I Avoid Becoming a Product Junkie?

How to Avoid Becoming a "Product Junkie" by Sticking to the Basics

With the widespread availability of natural products on the internet and even in local grocery stores, it takes some strong willpower to withstand the urge to start collecting products i.e. becoming a 'Product Junkie'.

If you start to notice that your bathroom shelves and cabinets are becoming over-crowed with natural hair products, not to mention the bank account getting thinner in the process, those are side effects of the "PJ syndrome".

One way to get rid of the "Product Junkie" syndrome is to commit to using at least 80% to 90% of the products you already have before purchasing new ones. Of course, this will be no easy feat due to the fact that it seems like every day there is a new testimony of a "wonderful, must-try" product advertised.

Below is a plan to help those who want to get rid of the PJ syndrome stick to this commitment. The plan is a simple one, but it is a sure way to keep you from becoming or staying a full blown Product Junkie.

The first thing to do is stick with staple products that fit into your hair care regimen. Something to clean your hair, condition your hair, seal in moisture and a styling agent - if anyone was counting that's a total of four products.

I know that for some just having four hair products in their arsenal may sound like an impossibility, but drastic times call for drastic measures. A cleansing agent, conditioner, moisturizer, and style agent are all anyone really needs to maintain their hair.

This plan even has room for a few allowances, maybe two product alternatives – bringing the total up to six if you want to switch up on different scents of a shampoo or moisturizer, add a leave-in conditioner, etc.

After you have narrowed down your staples, the next thing to do is to commit to using at least 80% to 90% of a product before replacing it. The reasoning behind not using 100% of a product is so you won't be caught in need of something and have none on hand before you get a chance to replenish.

How to Avoid Becoming a "Product Junkie" by Sticking to the Basics
continued

There will come a time or two when you are following this plan that you will have to battle PJ withdrawal. You will feel the urge to try something new that you've heard a great testimony about.

Of course, the 'plan' is not to buy anything until you finish the products you already have, but if the PJ monkey is jumping and pounding on your back there is a solution; only buy the sample-size of that product.

This will save you money, space, and if the product doesn't work with your hair texture you won't have a super-size bottle or jar just laying around. If there is not a sample size available, you will simply have to revert to waiting until you finish one of your older products to buy it. And of course, replace like products with like products i.e. a conditioner for a conditioner, etc.

Another thing to practice while on this plan is to use a set of products for an entire month, i.e. the same brand of shampoo, conditioner, moisturizer, etc. Depending on the size of products and/or the amount and frequency in which you use them, you may have to stretch this to two months at a time.

This will help you to avoid the thinning bank account side effect, because you won't just pick up products from every store you visit throughout the month since you have an entire set of products to use first.

Doing this will also help you to get a feel for a particular set of products as well, helping you figure out if they are actually worthy of repurchasing. Also, if you only wear certain styles in the summer, like wash-n-goes avoid buying products geared specifically for these styles year 'round.

In summary, sticking to basic staples, cleansing, conditioning, moisturizing and a styling product; using 80% to 90% of a product before buying a new one to replace it and replacing it with a like product; times when new products are screaming your name buying only sample-size products; and, avoiding buying products geared for seasonal styles, you will either be able to avoid becoming a Product Junkie, or be on your way to becoming a recovering Product Junkie.

Determining Safe Ingredients for Your Hair

With so many products on the market today proclaiming to be 'natural' it can be very confusing determining which ones are truly natural versus those that contain a few natural ingredients. And when it comes to reading ingredient lists, it seems like you need to be a chemist to understand them. For example, the average consumer might not know off hand that simmondsia chinensis is actually Jojoba.

The best way to determine whether a product is safe or not is to research its ingredients. Research sounds like a project, but with the help of the Internet it is actually quick and easy. A great site to conduct product and ingredient research is Skin Deep Cosmetic Safety Database. According to the website, Skin Deep gets about 1 million page views per month, and is the world's largest and most popular product safety guide.

Skin Deep is an online safety guide for cosmetics and personal care products that was launched in 2004 by the Environmental Working Group. Skin Deep's database provides safety ratings for nearly a quarter of all products on the market; 62,551 products with 7,644 ingredients. They also have a mobile app - EWG's Skin Deep.

Skin Deep ratings are on a 0 to 10 scale; 0 being low hazard and 10 being the highest. You can search ingredients, product brands, and even get a shopping list of low hazard products.

Just simply type in the entire product name or ingredient and you will get facts on the product/ingredient i.e. what it's used for, its rating, toxicity stats, as well as government and other agency studies performed. In a matter of minutes you will have all the information you need to determine whether or not you want to purchase a product, or stop using one you already have.

E. How Do I Make My Own Products?

Another way to save money on hair products is to make them yourself. You can become a 'Mixtress' or "Mixmeister" by making you own products from things that you already have in your kitchen. Need a conditioner? Try using mayonnaise, eggs, and/or yogurt.

Need a moisturizer? Break out that bottle of olive oil or jar of honey. How about a hair rinse that restores pH balance? Good old apple cider vinegar, with a dash of baking soda to combat itchiness will do.

By making your own products, you will be able to save money, keep your hair looking great and earn the bragging rights to say, "I made it myself."

DIY Temple Balm

Ponytails, updos, and buns are great cool summer styles. But these styles require the hair around the temples - edges - to be laid/slick down and/or stretched tightly back for a more polished look.

This can cause stress around the hairline. Too much stress that can be caused by tight braids and accessories as well as constantly pulling hair back can cause breakage along the hairline.

While ponytails, updos and buns do help with protecting our ends, our edges need pampering as well. There are several products available that proclaim to grow back or fill-in edges, but with a few simple ingredients, you can create your own.

The following list of ingredients will enable you to make a DIY temple balm, that will not only give your ponytails, updos and buns that 'polished' look, but will protect the hair around your temples, stimulate scalp circulation and promote hair growth.

The first step will be to decide whether you want an oil or pomade type balm. For an oil based balm, you can choose among the following carrier oils:

Jojoba Oil
Olive Oil
Coconut Oil
Hemp Oil
Neem Oil
Shea Oil
Sweet Almond Oil

For a pomade type balm you can choose among the following butters:

Cocoa Butter
Olive Butter
Aloe Butter
Hemp Butter
Shea Butter
Almond Butter

If you have a favorite carrier oil or butter that is not listed, you can use them as well

DIY Temple Balm *continued*

The next step will be to add essential oils and/or herbs to your oil or butter. Carrier oils can be infused with herbs. Essential oils can be added directly to your oils or butters. You can also add carrier oils infused with herbs to melted butter.

Essential Oils and Herbs

Arnica
Calendula
Stinging Nettle
Rosemary (oil or leaves)
Peppermint Oil
Sage (EO or leaves)
Cedarwood
Saw Palmetto Extract

For those who would prefer a gel type balm essential oils and/or infused carrier oils can be mixed with 3 parts Aloe Vera Gel and 1 part oil.

DIY Basic Temple Balm Recipe

Combine ¼ cup of carrier oil (see instruction link on Sources page if you want to make an herb infused oil), or butter in a 4 ounce container with 2 or more essential oils adding ¼ tsp of each. If you are using butter, melt butter before adding oils to make mixing easier, then let it sit to solidify. Feel free to tweak ingredients to your liking.

Use your temple balm as a hairdressing to smooth the edges when wearing ponytails, updos and buns, or just to protect and treat thinning edges. Your temple balm can also be used for scalp massages as well. For the 'polished' look, lightly moisturize your edges with water, then add your balm. Gently brush back and cover with a silk/satin scarf for approx. 20 to 30 mins or overnight.

Olive Oil

Olive oil seals in moisture, conditions, and improves the strength and elasticity of your hair; it also helps with dry, itchy scalp and kills head lice. Olive oil can be applied to dampened ends to seal in moisture as an effective way to prevent split ends. Mix olive oil with your favorite conditioner, and use it as a deep conditioning treatment.

Olive oil is the only vegetable oil that can be consumed as it is - freshly pressed from the fruit. It has a high content of monounsaturated fatty acids and antioxidative substances. Olive oil also protects against heart disease by controlling LDL cholesterol levels, while raising HDL cholesterol levels.

Store olive oil in a cool and dark place, tightly sealed, because when exposed to oxygen, light or high temperatures the oil can easily go rancid.

Recipes

Honey & Olive Oil Hair Mask
Mix ½ cup honey and 3 tablespoons olive oil. Work a small amount at a time through hair until coated. Cover hair with a shower cap; leave on 30 minutes. Shampoo well and rinse. Remember your final rinse should be done with cool water to close the hair cuticle.

Egg & Olive Oil Hair Mask
Mix two whole eggs with four tablespoons of olive oil. Smooth through hair. Wrap head with plastic wrap, and leave in hair for 10 minutes. Rinse well.

Olive Oil Hot Oil Treatment
Place ½ cup of olive oil in a bowl of boiling water (you can also pour the oil in an applicator bottle then sit it in a bowl of boiling water to warm). Massage the warm oil into your scalp and work your way to the ends. Cover your hair for 30 minutes with a shower cap and rinse. The warm oil penetrates more deeply into the hair shaft and will help repair damaged cuticles that cause dryness, frizziness and breakage.

Avocados for Healthy Hair

Avocados are not only beneficial to our bodies, providing over 20 essential nutrients which include potassium, fiber and Vitamins A and B, but they can also aid in healthy hair. Avocados, which are fruits by the way and not vegetables, have also been called alligator pears because of their shape and skin color. California produces about 90% of the nation's Avocado crop.

Avocados are rich in vitamins A, D and E, lecithin (a natural antioxidant, conditioner and moisturizer), beta-carotene (which converts to Vitamin A promoting healthy skin and nails) and more than 20% essential fatty acids. To prolong the life of your avocados, peel, seed and puree them, add a little lemon juice, put the mixture in an air-tight container and freeze. It will last up to four to five months before using.

Avocado oil is derived from the pulp of fresh avocados. Although the avocado is a fruit, its oil is categorized as a vegetable oil. The oil promotes the regeneration of scarred skin and softens and conditions dry, flaky skin and scalp. Avocado oil has a long shelf life (organic avocado oil lasts the longest).

Oil expressed from the flesh is rich in vitamins A, B, G and E. The oil contains vital amino acids such as oleic and linoleic, which are essential fatty acids that help eliminate eczema, psoriasis, dandruff, and aid in the prevention of hair loss.

Oleic is an omega nine fatty acid, rich in antioxidants which fight the side effects of free radicals, moisturizer and also aids in stronger and thicker hair growth. Linoleic is an omega three fatty acid, anti-inflammatory and promotes healthy hair growth. Both oleic and linoleic help in the absorption of Vitamins A, E and K, which work with essential fatty acids to provide healthy sheen to your hair and skin as well.

Avocado oil can be used to do scalp massages, as a pre-shampoo treatment, a hot oil treatment, and can even be added to your favorite conditioner to enhance its moisturizing properties.

Avocado Oil Shampoo
To prepare an avocado oil hair shampoo, you will need 1 teaspoon avocado oil, 1/2 teaspoon coconut or olive oil and 6 oz liquid castile soap. Mix all the ingredients together and store it in a bottle for at least 2 days to allow the ingredients to set. Use it to shampoo your hair on a regular basis.

Avocado Deep Conditioner

Peel, seed and mash one avocado and add 1 cup of coconut milk. Combine the ingredients together and mash until the mixture is smooth and thick. I strongly suggest you use a mixer for this or you will have bits and pieces of avocado in your hair that will take forever to rinse out.

Comb the mixture through your hair and wait about 10-15 minutes (you can also sit with a plastic cap on as well), then rinse off, making your final rinse with cool water.

Oily Hair Tips/Recipes

Seborrhoe, the medical term for oily hair occurs when the sebaceous glands, which are located at the base of each hair shaft, produce too much sebum. Oily hair can also be caused by poor hygiene and diet. There are several things you can do to combat oily hair.

Tips:

* Shampoo every other day.
* Rinse on the off day, add essential oils like lavender as a freshener. Remember to rinse with cool water to close the hair cuticles.
* Try to avoid using conditioner on your roots and scalp, instead concentrate on your ends.
* Avoid using styling products containing silicone. Don't brush your hair often, since brushing helps spread oil throughout your hair.
* Avoid fried and spicy foods. Consuming these stimulates our body's natural oil secretion causing oily hair to look even more oily and frizzy as a result. Add more vegetables to your diet.

At Home Recipes:

Shampoo Additions

1/2 teaspoon Aloe Vera gel (squeeze gel out of Aloe Vera plant) and 1 tablespoon lemon juice. Blend ingredients together with 1/4 cup of your regular hair shampoo. Wash hair then rinse well use cool water for your final rinse.

1/4 cup unscented mild, natural shampoo 1/4 cup sage tea, cooled and strained 15 drops cedarwood essential oil and 15 drops lavender essential oil. Combine all ingredients and shake well before using. Shampoo and rinse with cool water.

Dry Shampoo

To make a dry shampoo for oily hair, combine 1 tbsp. of cornstarch, 1 tbsp. of baking soda, and 1 tbsp. of dry oatmeal. Blend together in a food processor or blender until very fine. Take 1 tsp. of this mixture, bend over a sink with your hair hanging forward, and apply the powder mixture into your scalp near the roots. Gently massage into the scalp and hair. Brush out the dry shampoo thoroughly.

Hair Rinses:

Tea and Lemon Rinse
Brew tea (sage, chamomile, tea tree, eucalyptus) and add the juice of two
fresh lemons (you can substitute with lemon juice). Let cool and massage
on scalp and leave on for 20 mins to 30 mins and rinse with cool water.
This rinse can even be left in.

Vinegar Rinse
2 teaspoons of white vinegar and ¼ cup of water. Massage on scalp and
leave on for ½ hour and rinse. You actually do not have to rinse this if you
use more water and less vinegar - about one cap-full to one cup of water.

Natural Herbs That Promote Hair Growth

There are several products lining beauty supply shelves that promise hair growth, but all in all, hair growth is not achieved by a 'magic' or 'miracle' product. Age, genetics and diet are all factors in hair length, but, on average, our hair grows about a quarter to a half an inch a month.

Although there is not one product that can make hair grow faster, there are several natural herbs and ingredients that stimulate the scalp and aid in hair growth.

Aloe

Aloe can be applied directly onto your scalp and promotes hair growth. It stimulates blood circulation in the scalp and also fights against alopecia.

Horsetail contains high concentrations of silicic acid and other silicates. It also contains potassium, aluminum, and manganese, all of which aid in the prevention of hair loss.

How to Use: Boil a handful of horsetail leaves with stems in a gallon of water. Let the horsetail sit for about 20-25 minutes and then use the water as the last rinse after washing hair. You can also **buy the herb in capsule form**.

CAUTION: EXCESSIVE USE OF HORSETAIL HERB COULD LEAD TO DRYNESS IN HAIR OR DERMATITIS.

Evening Primrose, Stinging Nettle & Rosemary

Evening Primrose increases blood circulation in the hair follicle and is high in the essential fatty acid known as gamma-linolenic acid which stimulates hair growth. You can purchase Evening Primrose in both capsule and oil.

Stinging nettle disinfects the scalp and increases blood circulation. It blocks the enzymes that cause hair loss and promotes hair re-growth.

Rosemary stimulates the scalp and helps prevent dry scalp and dandruff. It is also a natural hair conditioner.

Rosemary Hair Rinse

Boil rosemary leaves in one cup of water and let steep for 5 to 7 minutes. After cooling, use the liquid as a final rinse after washing, or pour into a spray bottle as a daily leave-in. Keep the mixture refrigerated and add a few drops of sage as a preservative if you are planning to keep the mixture longer than one week.

Sage

Sage is a stimulant and is anti-bacterial. Sage essential oil can be combined with rosemary and lavender and used on your scalp. This will help to balance the oils in your scalp and help stimulate hair growth.

Sage Tea and Apple Cider Vinegar

Apple cider vinegar has a very high natural pH and gets rid of product build-up by dissolving minerals, toxins, and dirt particles as well as fights dry scalp and dandruff.

Scalp Treatment

Mix four ounces of apple cider vinegar (ACV) with four ounces of cooled sage tea or ten drops of sage essential oil. Pour the mixture on your scalp, then wrap your hair with a towel or put on a plastic cap for 20 to 30 minutes. Rinse and shampoo as usual.

After Wash Rinse

Add about 5 drops of sage oil, or 2 cups of cooled sage tea, with 1 capful of ACV and use as a final rinse after washing. The mixture does not have to be washed out.

Honey Recipes

Honey naturally attracts and holds moisture. It is also a natural antiseptic and contains antioxidants. Honey is packed with vitamins and minerals such as magnesium, potassium, calcium, sulphur, iron, zinc and vitamins B1, B2, B3, which aid in hair growth. It can be added to conditioners, rinses and pomades.

Most of the honey hair recipes I've come across contain a mix of honey and olive oil. Try using this honey (pre-poo) treatment. Mix honey and olive oil in equal parts, distribute on hair, put on your shower cap and let sit for 30 minutes before rinsing and washing.

Brown Sugar Hair and Scalp Cleaner from Nappy Kitchen.com (website no longer active): 1 tablespoon of brown sugar and 3 tablespoons of your favorite conditioner. Mix ingredients together, wet your hair and scalp. Use your fingertips (NOT NAILS) to massage scalp in small circles. Rinse well. Use cool water on the last rinse, for shine.

Honey & Olive Oil Conditioner also from Nappy Kitchen.com. 1 tablespoon of honey, 1/2 teaspoon of extra virgin olive oil, and 1 cup warm water. Mix honey and olive oil well. Add to water and stir well. Distribute evenly over your hair. Apply plastic cap for 15 to 20 minutes. Rinse well and style as usual.

Honey Hair Conditioner

Mix 2 Tablespoons of honey with 1/2 of a fresh avocado and 1 Teaspoon of coconut oil. Massage into hair and leave on for half an hour. This works beautifully for dry and damaged hair.

Pre-wash treatment from Deecoily of Nappturality.com - it should be used before shampooing to condition the scalp and repair damaged hair. She suggests that you use it regularly if your hair is dry or ends are split. You will need 2 tablespoons of olive oil, 2 teaspoons of honey, 5 drops rosemary, lavender or geranium essential oil, a small cup, a ceramic or glass bowl, a small stainless steel spoon, a plastic shower cap and a comfortably hot towel.

In a cup sitting in hot water, warm the olive oil and honey (or use the microwave but be careful not to burn yourself). Stir in your choice of essential oil and mix well. While the mixture is still warm, apply it all over your hair, massaging well into your scalp.

Honey Recipes *continued*

Cover your hair with the shower cap (or large plastic bag) and wrap the towel around your head and leave on for 10-15 minutes. For severely damaged hair, she suggests that you leave the mixture on up to 30 minutes. Remove the towel and shower cap, and wash your hair with a mild or baby shampoo.

I mix honey in my final rinse after shampooing. I use two to three cups of tea (I use green tea, but you can use your favorite, you may also need to increase the amount of water depending on your hair length), one teaspoon of melted honey (if you add more water, use 1 tablespoon), one tablespoon of lemon juice.

After making the tea, add the honey and mix well, then add the lemon juice. Remember to let the mixture cool before pouring over your hair and do not rinse. I follow with a leave-in conditioner and style. A tablespoon of ACV - apple cider vinegar - can also be added to this mixture.

Dyeing and Conditioning with Henna

You can dye your hair naturally with Henna. Henna is a flowering plant, and its scientific name is Lawsonia inermis.

Henna produces a red/orange dye molecule called lawsone. Lawsone, is primarily concentrated in the leaves, and is in the highest levels in the petioles of the leaf.

This molecule has an affinity for bonding with protein and has been used to dye skin, hair, fingernails, leather, silk and wool. When using henna to dye hair, lawsone binds with keratin located in the hair shaft.

Henna's whole leaves will not stain the skin until the lawsone molecules are released from the henna leaf. Dried, ground, sifted henna leaves can be worked into a paste that can be used to make body art henna.

The powder can be then mixed with lemon juice, strong tea, or other mildly acidic liquids. Essential oils such as tea tree, eucalyptus or lavender can be also added, all of which will improve the stain characteristics.

Then the henna mix must rest for 6 to 12 hours so the leaf cellulose is dissolved, and thus releases more dye. Body art henna is great for dyeing hair because the powder rinses out easier (even out of braids and locs) and the color is richer. Body art henna is safe to use over dyed, bleached, and permed hair.

Be aware that henna comes in one color. There are several commercial henna hair dyes on the market that come in various colors, but they are not 100% pure henna because chemicals are added.

The color you will get when dyeing your hair with henna depends on your natural hair color. Henna on natural dark hair doesn't dye it red, but gives it red highlights, and over time improves shine and helps repair damage from chemicals.

The natural dyeing process of henna takes about four days. During this time the lawsone is binding to the keratin molecule. As the days go by, the darker your hair will get, especially if you mixed the powder with an acidic liquid like lemon juice. Repeated applications will result in richer, deeper color.

Dyeing and Conditioning with Henna *continued*

Through CurlyNikki.com, I learned of the site Henna For Hair. Among the information on the Henna for Hair site are henna fact pages, a Henna Encyclopedia, YouTube 'how to' videos, a henna forum, a Mehandi shop where you can purchase henna, and other products.

The site also has a free downloadable Henna "How To" ebook. The ebook covers such topics as, "What is Henna?', "How do you dye your hair with henna?" pictures, and a quick mix reference chart.

In the picture on the cover of this book you can see the results of henna on my hair. The red streak (which used to be gray) is the result of my once-a-month henna treatments.

HennaSooq.com is my favorite place to purchase henna. The look on the cover was created with their Red Raj henna, mixed with 3 tablespoons of their Organic Hibiscus Petal Powder, green tea, 1 tablespoon of Grapeseed oil and 1 tablespoon of honey.

DIY Healthy Hair Beverages

One of the latest trends for overall health is juicing. Those who are picky about eating certain fruits and vegetables are finding it easier to drink them. Juicing is not only a great way to get our recommended daily fruit and vegetable intake, but also a great way to nourish our bodies from the inside out.

By blending a few simple fruits and vegetables you can also juice your way to healthy hair (of course, exercise plays a role as well). Also by adding a little ice to your ingredients, or even using frozen fruits and vegetables you can turn your juices into smoothies. With no specific recipe needed, there are a variety of fruits and vegetables that can be blended together that both aid in hair and overall body health.

Fruits that aid in healthy hair ...

Fruit and/or real fruit juice will add some sweetness to your drink. Blueberries are packed with vitamin C which is very helpful when it comes to circulation to the scalp and blood vessels that nourish the hair follicles. The lack of vitamin C in your diet can lead to hair breakage.

Citrus fruits such as oranges, limes, grapefruits and lemons are great sources of vitamin C. Likewise, adding fruits like pineapples, nectarines and cantaloupe which are high in beta-carotene converts vitamin A in our bodies, which helps produce oils that aid in the health of our scalp. The lack of vitamin A can result in itchiness and dandruff.

Along with blueberries, raspberries and strawberries are also high in vitamin B which provides cells with oxygen which helps reduce hair loss and stimulates hair growth.

Bananas are another great fruit that can be added to your juices or smoothies. They are packed with nutrients including vitamins A, B, C and E along with minerals like potassium, zinc, iron and manganese. Potassium is known to help in increasing blood circulation in the body which leads to healthy skin and aides in hair growth. Potassium, iron, zinc and manganese deficiencies can result in hair loss.

DIY Healthy Hair Beverages *continued*

Veggies that aid in healthy hair ...

Carrots can also be added to your juice. They are a good source of vitamin A, which helps promote overall hair and scalp health. Carrots also help with healthy sebum production, which can lead to faster hair growth. They also help keep hair shiny and conditioned.

Dark leafy-green vegetables such as spinach make great juices and/or smoothies. Spinach is packed with iron, beta-carotene, folate (both helpful in hair growth) and vitamin C that promote healthy hair follicles and help circulate scalp oils. Dark leafy-green vegetables are composed of disease - fighting phytochemicals, as well as antioxidants that fight free radicals (that can cause tissue and cell damage) and help to strengthen hair.

They also contain a very high percentage of water, which helps keep your hair and skin properly hydrated, without which, your skin and hair begin to look dry. Broccoli, kale and Swiss chard can also be used to make healthy hair drinks.

Adding some Greek yogurt to your dark leafy-green vegetables for juicing will help with hair health as well. Greek yogurt is high in protein, vitamin B5 (pantothenic acid) which promotes hair growth, and vitamin D.

You see it's just as simple as that; by combining a leafy-green vegetable such as spinach or kale, some Greek yogurt and a few slices of fruit and blending them together you will not only have a nutritious juice or smoothie, but a healthy drink that will aid in the overall health of your hair.

III

The 10 Natural Hair Commandments

I – Thou shalt be thankful for the hair that adorns thy head. Your hair is your 'crown of glory' treat it as such.

II – Thou shalt not idolize the hair that adorns another's head. The hair on your head is unique, it's what makes you you.

III – Thou shalt not take the hair that adorns thy head in vain. Be aware of the damage that chemicals and heat can cause, some of the damage is irreversible.

IV – Remember to take the necessary time to pamper thy hair. Create a routine, set aside specific days for sealing your ends, massaging, trimming, washing, conditioning and styling your hair. A healthy head of hair will be your reward.

V – Honor thy mother, father and ancestors for the beautiful traits that they have bestowed upon thee, one of which is your natural crown of glory. Wear your natural hair with pride.

VI – Thou shalt not attempt to use a fine-tooth comb to detangle thy hair. Even before using a wide-tooth comb, use your fingers to detangle, and when detangling always start from the ends and work your way up towards your scalp.

VII – Thou shalt not be ashamed to wear your natural hair in public. Wigs, weaves, braid extensions etc. are all wonderful temporary 'protective' and 'transition' styles, but they don't compare to the beauty of your natural hair.

VIII – Thou shalt not kill the hair follicles on thy head – with high heat, harsh chemicals or tight styles. Stay away from pore clogging, dry scalp causing petroleum based products; use natural essential oil based ones instead. Be gentle with your hair, seek out professional stylists who have experience in styling your hair type.

IX – Thou shalt not bad mouth thy neighbor's hair. Be respectful and encouraging to those who have not yet chosen to wear their hair natural. Negative comments will only turn them away from the natural hair community.

The 10 Natural Hair Commandments *continued*

X – Thou shalt not covet thy neighbor's hair; thou shalt not covet its texture, nor its curl pattern, or its length, etc. Appreciate the hair that you were blessed with. Try different styles and accessories that accentuate your very own personality and style.

IV

Sources

Transitioning Movement
Black History.com
NY Times.com
Naturally Isis.com
Melissa Harris-Perry Show – MHPHSHOW.MSNBC.MSN.com

Resisting Hair Growth Remedies
WebMD.com - Minoxidil
UK Medix.com - Hair Loss Remedies
Live Strong.com – Natural Ways to Promote Hair Growth

Preventing Split Ends
More information on split ends:
www.devon-trichology-practice.co.uk/hair.asp
www.ultimate-cosmetics.com/beauty/hair-care/split-ends.htm

Consider Ayurvedic Natural Hair Care
Ayurvedic Approach to Beauty - www.ayurbalance.com
Ayurveda Info - www.bluelotusayurveda.com
Ayurveda Resources - www.umm.edu
Ayurvedic Hair Recipes - www.ayurveda-herbal-remedy.com
Ayurvedic Clarifying Rinse – www.ehow.com – Make Tea Clarifying Hair Rinse
Article on Ayurvedic Health/Hair Care - www.cocoandcreme.com
Free Dosha Quiz - www.whatsyourdosha.com

Determining Safe Ingredients for Your Hair
Skin Deep Cosmetic Safety Database - www.cosmeticsdatabase.com
Skin Deep App – EWG's Skin Deep

DIY Temple Balm
Visit AnniesRemedy.com for infusing oil instructions
Purchase Ingredients
FromNatureWithLove.com
MountainRoseHerbs.com
NewDirectionsAromatics.com

Sources *continued*

Olive Oil
Olive Oil Source.com
Healing Daily.com
Health Recipes.com
Olives 101.com

Avocados for Hair
Avocado Oil Recipes - www.buzzle.com
Avocado Info -www.hort.purdue.edu
Avocado.org

Oily Hair
Go Herbal Remedies.com

Natural Herbs for Hair Growth
Pioneer Thinking.com
eHow.com - Horsetail Recipe
StopHairloss.com

Honey Recipes
Nappturality.com
eHow.com

Dyeing and Conditioning with Henna
Henna for Hair.com
Henna Encyclopedia -
www.hennapage.com/henna/encyclopedia/index.html
Free Henna 'How-To' book - www.hennaforhair.com/freebooks/
Henna on Wikipedia.org
Henna Page.com
Mehandi.com
Laquita's Favorite Place to Purchase Henna – www.hennasooq.com

Natural Hair Certification Classes/Styling Services
Madam Walker's Braids & Lockery, Temple Hills, MD
www.madamwalkersbraids.com